Fundamentals of Nursing

Master Nursing School and the NCLEX® Exam
110 Practice Test Questions with Rationales

Anna Curran, RN, BSN, PHN

Disclaimer

Every effort has been made to ensure that the information in this guide is correct. The publisher and author do not assume and hereby disclaim any liability to any party for any loss, disruption, or damage caused by errors and omissions, whether such errors or omissions result from accident, negligence, or any other cause.

This book is not intended as a substitute for the medical advice of physicians. The reader should regularly consult with a physician in matters relation to his or her health and particularly with respect to any signs and symptoms that may require diagnosis or medical attention.

About The Author

Anna Curran, RN, BSN, PHN

Emergency Room Registered Nurse

Critical Care Transport Nurse

Clinical Nurse Instructor for LVN and BSN students

Anna began writing materials to help her BSN and LVN students with their studies. She takes the topics that the students are learning and expands on them to try to help with their understanding of the nursing process. Her experience spans over two decades in nursing, starting as an LVN in 1993. She received her RN license in 1997. She has worked in Medical-Surgical, Telemetry, ICU and the ER. She found a passion in the ER and has stayed in this department for 16 years. She is a clinical instructor for LVN and BSN students, along with a critical care transport nurse.

Thanks again for downloading this book. If you like the book, please leave us feedback and let us know.

Fundamentals Review Questions without Answers and Rationales
NCLEX: Fundamentals of Nursing

1. An elderly patient is admitted under your care and exhibits an impaired gait. To reduce the risk of falls, to which member of the healthcare team should you refer this patient?

    A. Nurse practitioner

    B. Podiatrist

    C. Occupational therapist

    D. Physical therapist

2. Your hospital uses the SBAR reporting system to relay information between the members of the healthcare team. Which of the following includes the correct elements of SBAR?

    A. Signs and Symptoms, Basic patient information, Action, and Reaction

    B. Situation, Background, Action, and Recommendation

C. Situation, Background, Assessment, and Recommendation

D. Signs and Symptoms, Background, Action, and Reaction

3. A patient complains of having a burning sensation and pain on the peripheral cannula site. You observe that there is warmth, redness, swelling and tenderness on the area. The patient is likely to be suffering from:

A. Phlebitis
B. Infiltration
C. Hematoma
D. Infection

4. A healthcare provider is about to render personal care to a 77-year old patient. It is important to use long and firm strokes and start from distal to proximal areas in order to:

A. Preserve the skin integrity
B. Reduce the risk of blood clot
C. Increase venous blood return
D. Promote vasoconstriction

5. A terminal patient under your care had peacefully died 10 minutes ago. While you prepare to inform the patient's family of the event, it is important to note which of the following five stages of death and dying according to Kubler-Ross?

A. Bereavement, Crying, Depression, Regret, Denial
B. Anger, Bargaining, Denial, Depression, Acceptance
C. Bereavement, Anger, Denial, Depression, Acceptance
D. Anger, Regret, Bereavement, Loneliness, Depression

6. A 65-year old patient is suspected to have hypoxia. Which of the following diagnostic tests should be done to verify this?

A. Full blood count
B. Biochemistry
C. Arterial Blood Gas (ABG) Analysis
D. Hemoglobin level

7. A 35-year old patient is being monitored for adverse reactions to barbiturate therapy. One of these is considered as a major disadvantage of barbiturate therapy.

   A. Hepatotoxicity
   B. Drug dependence
   C. Reduced absorption
   D. Slow action

8. A 78 –year old female patient has severe difficulty of swallowing. The doctor and the dietitian agreed to prescribe enteral feeding for her. Which of the following nursing actions should be done when giving continuous enteral feeding?

   A. Warm the enteral feed formula using a microwave
   B. Elevate the head of the bed
   C. Ask the patient to lean on her left side
   D. Administer at a standard rate of 100 mL per hour

9. A post-mastectomy patient arrives in the surgical unit for continuity of care. After 4 hours, the nurse comes into the patient's room and suspects that she might be having shock as evidenced by:

A. Pale, dry, and warm skin

B. Urine output of 30 mL per hour

C. Respiratory rate of 17

D. Restlessness

10. A nurse working in an outpatient unit witnesses a 65-year old male patient to faint and become unconscious. During rapid assessment, which pulse should the nurse palpate?

A. Femoral

B. Carotid

C. Radial

D. Brachial

11. A nurse is caring for a pregnant patient who is at a very high risk for a life-threatening situation while her baby is also at high risk for fetal death. Which of the following roles should the nurse prioritize?

A. Advocate

B. Coordinator of care

C. Case manager

D. Collaborator

12. In the emergency room, a 44-year old male patient agrees to be admitted in the medical after the physician diagnosed him with lower respiratory tract infection. He sits on the wheelchair and the porter brings him to the ward. Which type of legal consent was exhibited?

   A. Explicit consent
   B. Opt-out consent
   C. Implicit consent
   D. Emergency consent

13. A newly diagnosed Parkinson's patient suffers from hand tremors. She will need adaptive devices to help her cut food and eat her meals properly. The nurse can refer this patient to which member of the multidisciplinary healthcare team?

   A. Physical therapist
   B. Occupational therapist
   C. Dietitian
   D. Nutritionist

14. A 74-year old male patient with congestive heart failure was admitted in the Intensive Care Unit. After 10 days, his condition has stabilized and he is now to be transferred to the medical ward. Which of the following terms best describes this scenario?

    A. Critical pathway
    B. Continuity of Care
    C. Case Management
    D. Cardiac protocol

15. A community health nurse is planning a presentation on the risk factors for cancer. Which of the following categories of risk factors is considered the most modifiable?

    A. Lifestyle choices
    B. External locus of control
    C. Genetic predisposition
    D. High risk behaviors

16. A nurse needs to relay important information to the patient's attending physician. Which of the following

statements should be included in the "Assessment" part of SBAR?

A. The nurse tells the doctor that the patient's current diagnosis is ulcerative colitis.
B. The nurse informs the physician that the patient has 3 episodes of watery stools.
C. The nurse tells the doctor that the patient may benefit from additional IV fluids.
D. The nurse informs the physician that the stool culture is positive for C. difficile.

17. A post-surgical male patient is about to be discharged. The nurse shows the home medications that the patient needs to take and tells him the right doses and frequency for each drug. The nurse asks the patient to repeat the information back to her to assess his understanding. Which of the following professional roles does the nurse perform in this scenario?

A. Advocate
B. Case manager
C. Care giver
D. Educator

18. A female patient is going to have a hysterectomy in the afternoon. She shows the early signs of heightened anxiety. Which of the following is the best response by the healthcare provider?

   A. "Here's a booklet on your procedure. Read it and let me know if you have any questions."
   B. "Would you like me to turn on the television to distract you while waiting for the surgery?"
   C. "What is bothering you regarding this surgery?
   D. "Everything will be okay, so don't worry too much about it."

19. A patient complains of abdominal pain. The nurse starts the assessment with which of the following examination techniques?

   A. Percussion
   B. Auscultation
   C. Palpation
   D. Inspection

20. A patient starting on chemotherapy has recently had a central venous catheter inserted for optimal access. In checking the radiological report on the proper positioning of this catheter, the tip should be in the:

A. Subclavian vein
B. Superior vena cava
C. Basilica vein
D. Jugular vein

21. During the night shift, an 83-year old female patient complains of not being able to sleep. Which of the following nursing interventions should the nurse do first?

A. Assist the client with the use of sleep aids such as pillows, snacks, back rubs, and a change of room temperature as needed.
B. Ask the physician to prescribe a sleeping medication and administer it.
C. Educate the patient to perform deep breathing exercises, guided imagery, and relaxation techniques.
D. Assess the patient's sleeping patterns and record in her sleeping chart.

22. A 45-year old male patient is rushed into the emergency room following a serious motor vehicle accident. Which of the following nursing actions should the nurse prioritize?

   A. Administer pain relief
   B. Use a pillow as a splint to the chest wall
   C. Assess the patient's airway
   D. Teach the patient to perform deep breathing exercises

23. A 66-year old female patient goes back to the surgical ward after having a tonsillectomy. After 2 hours, the patient exhibits signs of lethargy and sore throat. Which of the following positions should be encouraged?

   A. Side-lying
   B. High Fowler's
   C. Supine
   D. Semi Fowler's

24. A nurse needs to conduct a client interview on the patient's past medical history and current medications.

Which of the following is the most appropriate behavior during the interview?

A. Sit on the chair at the bedside of the client and use active listening
B. Ask the patient, "Why did you choose to be admitted this time?"
C. Use accurate medical terms when asking questions
D. Provide a medical interview form to the patient, and come back when he/she has already finished answering it

25. A 24-year old male patient is newly admitted in the medical ward and the nurse attempts to do an initial set of vital signs for him. What is the best position of the patient for this assessment, considering that there are no contraindications?

A. Side-lying
B. Supine
C. Prone
D. Sitting upright

26. The nurse is performing a physical assessment of a 44-year old colitis patient. Which of the following will the nurse auscultate for when using the diaphragm of the stethoscope?

    A. Carotid bruits
    B. Heart murmurs
    C. Jugular venous hums
    D. Bowel sounds

27. A 22-year old female patient's body mass index is calculated as 27. This BMI can be considered as:

    A. Underweight
    B. Overweight
    C. Obese
    D. Average

28. The nurse is identifying some possible nursing diagnoses for a 32-year old post mastectomy patient. Which of the following models can she use to perform this?

Select all that apply

    A. Gordon's functional health patterns

B. Body systems model

C. Maslow's hierarchy of needs

D. Head-to-toe physical assessment form

29. A patient who is morbidly obese will benefit from reducing the pressure from the skin folds using which of the following nursing interventions?

A. Applying barrier cream on the skin

B. Using a sheepskin mattress protector

C. Aiding the skin folds with towels

D. Keeping the linens wrinkle free

30. A nurse is doing a physical assessment of an 82-year old female patient. The assessment revealed that she has all of the following secondary defenses against infection, except:

A. Swelling of lymph nodes

B. Intact skin

C. Pus on the infected wound

D. Fever

31. A patient is recovering from a massive stroke and exhibits signs of difficulty of swallowing. The nurse needs to refer this patient to which member of the multidisciplinary healthcare team?

    A. Physical therapist
    B. Speech therapist
    C. Respiratory therapist
    D. Occupational therapist

32. A 50-year old male patient has an established ascending colostomy. Before changing the colostomy bag, the nurse assesses the site and is likely to inform the physician about which of the following findings?

    A. The colostomy delivered liquid feces.
    B. There is redness on the skin after immediately removing the appliance.
    C. The stoma is raised to ½ inch above the abdomen.
    D. The stoma has a purplish color.

33. A 49-year old female patient calls for a nurse in her room and complains of abdominal pain and is also worried about her stools. Upon assessment, the nurse will suspect of

intestinal bleeding with which of the following stool characteristics?

    A. Watery and greenish stools

    B. Yellow blobs of stool floating in the toilet

    C. Soft and black, tarry stools

    D. Pencil shaped brown stools

34. An elderly female patient had a hip surgery following a fall and now shows signs of fecal incontinence. The nurse can use which of the following nursing diagnoses? Select all that apply.

    A. Disturbed Body Image

    B. Risk for deficient fluid volume

    C. Bowel incontinence

    D. Risk for impaired skin integrity

35. A nurse manager shows a new male nurse around the unit and shows the different equipment used for personal care. She tells him that a fracture bedpan can be used for which kind of patient?

    A. On bedrest

B. Dementia

C. Morbidly obese

D. Has a spinal cord injury

36. A female nurse is discussing effective ways to manage constipation with a 65-year old patient. She tells the patient to avoid excessive straining when trying to pass stools to prevent:

A. Fecal impaction
B. Dysrhythmia
C. Incontinence
D. Hemorrhoids

37. The nurse instructs the patient on how to properly collect a stool sample for a stool culture test. Which of the following should be included in this teaching?

A. The stool specimen must not be mixed with any drop of urine.
B. The sample bottle must be filled to the top.
C. Eating a lot of meat prior to stool collection is optimal.
D. If the stool is red in color, it is unacceptable.

38. A nurse notices that the patient with chronic obstructive pulmonary disease (COPD) has bluish discoloration of the lips. What the accurate term that she should use when documenting this finding?

A. Dyspnea
B. Cyanosis
C. Hypoxia
D. Hypoxemia

39. A patient with upper respiratory tract infection is unable to remove his phlegm on his own. The nurse uses a nasopharyngeal suction using which appropriate technique?

A. Hyper-oxygenate the patient with 100% oxygen for 30 minutes
B. Rotate the catheter while suctioning
C. Suction intermittently while inserting the catheter
D. Lubricate the catheter generously with petroleum jelly

40. A patient who has chronic pulmonary disease needs teaching on how to use the incentive spirometer properly. Which of the following statements indicate correct understanding of this procedure?

  A. "I can use the device three times a day before and after meals. "
  B. "I should breathe in fast and breathe out as fast and hard as I can."
  C. "I must inhale in a slowly and steady manner in order to keep the balls up."
  D. "I should use soapy water to clean the device every week."

41. A nurse conducts health teaching on the patient who is post hip replacement surgery. She tells the patient that the best way to implement deep breathing exercises includes which of the following?

  A. Use diaphragmatic breathing with pursed lips 5 to 10 times a day
  B. Perform forceful coughing 3 to 5 times a day
  C. Conduct deep breathing exercises 1 hour before and after meals

D. Use huff coughing every 2 hours or as the patient can tolerate

42. A 6-year old patient requires tracheostomy care. before starting to perform the procedure the first thing that the nurse should do includes:

A. Clean the incision site
B. Ask the patient to raise his right hand if he feels any pain or distress while doing the procedure
C. Change the twill tape that holds the tracheostomy in place
D. Check how tied the knot and ties are

43. The patient verbalizers, "I feel short of breath when I'm lying down, but I seem to feel better when I sit upright." The nurse recognizes that the patient is experiencing:

A. Acapnea
B. Orthopnea
C. Hypernea
D. Dyspnea

44. A 44-year old patient is diagnosed with acute bronchitis. The physician ordered to start corticosteroid therapy. The nurse tells the patient that corticosteroids will help:

    A. Facilitate coughing
    B. Achieve bronchodilation
    C. Reduce the inflammation of the airways
    D. Avoid contracting a respiratory infection

45. A male patient with chronic pulmonary disease is unable to expectorate phlegm on her own. The nurse plans to do postural drainage and percussion to help him. When is the best time for the nurse to do this procedure?

    A. After breakfast so the patient has energy
    B. Before lunch with an empty stomach
    C. 30 minutes after hyper-oxygenating the patient
    D. After dinner so the patient can sleep right after the procedure

46. A male elderly patient is prescribed with intravenous therapy and requires a new peripheral cannula to be inserted on his forearm. Because of a previous difficulty in

cannulation, the nurse decides to apply a warm compress on the forearm prior to doing the procedure. The nurse explains to the patient that the heat:

A. Alleviates the discomfort
B. Minimizes the muscle spasms
C. Increases circulation
D. Prevents hemorrhage

47. The doctor refers a newly admitted 85-year old female patient to chest physiotherapy service with the goal of expectorating thick phlegm using vibration and percussion. With the correct knowledge of the patient's past medical history, the nurse needs to question this order if the patient has:

A. Cystic fibrosis
B. Osteoporosis
C. Emphysema
D. Bronchitis

48. A male patient calls the nurse and complains of difficulty of breathing. He is already receiving oxygen via

nasal cannula while lying in bed. What is the first nursing intervention that must be performed?

A. Notify the physician
B. Check for any secretions and suction as needed
C. Assist the patient to a Fowler's position
D. Assess the oxygen levels using a pulse oximeter

49. An 89-year old nursing home resident gets admitted to the medical unit after 4 days of refusing to eat or drink. Which of the following findings should the health care provider expect?

A. Swollen mucous membranes
B. Distention of the jugular veins
C. High blood pressure
D. Weak and rapid pulse

50. A 60-year old male patient comes into the emergency unit with nausea and dizziness, and has had 5 episodes of watery, loose stools. Upon assessment, the patient verbalizes, "I've been having leg cramps since last night and I feel so weak." Which nursing intervention must be done first?

A. Administer an anti-emetic drug.

B. Review the patient's serum electrolytes.

C. Start an intravenous drip.

D. Ask the doctor to prescribe pain medication for leg cramping.

51. A nurse teaches the patient on proper breathing exercises. When teaching the patient about the purpose of pursed lip breathing, the nurse should inform the patient that it helps:

A. Lower intrathoracic pressure

B. Facilitate more effective coughing

C. Help keep the airways open

D. Allow the patient to expectorate phlegm

52. A senior staff nurse teaches a student nurse on the principles of precautions in the medical unit. The nurse tells the student to use clean gloves in which of the following nursing interventions for a non-isolated patient?

A. Performing oral care

B. Doing a back rub

C. Assisting the client in feeding

D. Providing hair care

53. A 75-year old male patient is admitted due to severe dehydration, diarrhea and vomiting. Which is the best method of assessing the patient's temperature?

A. Axillary
B. Oral
C. Radial
D. Tympanic

54. Upon doing baseline observations, the nurse records the respiratory rate of the patient as 25 respirations per minute in room air. Which of the following terms is appropriate in documenting this finding?

A. Hyperpyrexia
B. Tachypnea
C. Tachycardia
D. Arrhythmia

55. A nurse is doing a neurological examination on a newly admitted patient. Using the Glasgow Coma Scale, the patient scores 15 out of 15. This means that the patient is:

A. Unconscious
B. Semi-conscious
C. Fully alert
D. Has a minor brain injury

56. A patient with a Glasgow Coma Scale (GCS) score of 5 requires frequent mouth care. Before starting the procedure, the nurse should position the patient:

A. Trendelenburg
B. Lithotomy
C. Fowler's
D. Side lying

57. A 92-year old patient is newly admitted to the medical-surgical unit. Upon assessment, the nurse indicates that the patient is at high risk for falls because of all of the following factors except:

A. History of allergic rhinitis

B. Advanced age

C. Recent hip fracture

D. Use of a cane

58. A 36-year old female patient comes into the emergency unit with complaints of nausea, vomiting, abdominal cramping, and watery stools. The nurse asks the patient some questions regarding any recent food intake. Which of the following phases of nursing process does this scenario show?

A. Assessment

B. Diagnosis

C. Planning

D. Implementation

59. A medical-surgical nurse wants to apply Orem's theory in the nursing plan of care for a female patient with severe pulmonary disease. Which of the following can the nurse include in the care plan?

A. Love and belongingness

B. Physiological needs

C. Maintenance of sufficient intake of air

D. Self-perception

60. An elderly patient with full mental capacity refuses an injection, but the nurse administers the injection anyway as he/she thinks the patient needs it urgently. The nurse has committed:

A. Malpractice
B. Negligence
C. Assault and battery
D. None of the above

61. A 25-month old pediatric patient comes into the emergency unit with fever, irritability, dry lips, and watery loose stools. The mother said that the child has had 3 episodes of water loose stools since the previous night. After assessing the patient, the nurse should prioritize which of the following interventions?

A. Check the skin turgor

B. Obtain venous access

C. Weight the patient

D. Administer anti-diarrhea medication

62. Upon performing a physical assessment of a newly admitted female patient, the patient shows a positive Homan's sign. Which of the following nursing interventions is the highest priority of the nurse?

A. Promote patient's skin integrity

B. Promote venous circulation

C. Maintain patency of the airways

D. Improve the balance of fluids and electrolytes

63. A terminally ill cancer patient tells the nurse, "I am so afraid. Everyday my life seems to go downhill" The nurse responds, "Tell me more about how you're feeling." What kind of therapeutic technique is being used?

A. Sympathy

B. Exploring

C. Focusing

D. Acknowledgement

64. An 89-yearold male patient with stage IV lung cancer is about to start on chemotherapy. He tells

the nurse, "I don't actually want to have chemotherapy, but my children really want me to get this

treatment." The nurse should assume which of the following professional roles to protect this

patient?

A. Client advocate

B. Care provider

C. Educator

D. Counselor

65. A burn patient comes into the medical unit and shows signs of dehydration and blood loss. To encourage hydration, which of the following intravenous fluids should the nurse recommend to the

physician?

A. Lactated Ringer's solution

B. 0.9% Sodium Chloride

C. Dextrose 5% in Normal Saline

D. Dextrose 5% in Water

66. An occupational health nurse is planning a short seminar on stress and its effect to employees.

The nurse recognizes that stress can be described as all of the following except:

A. Stress may be physical, emotional, and/or spiritual.

B. Stress is a natural response and can be both adaptive and productive

C. Stress does not always lead to bodily damage

D. Stress always leads to feeling of hopelessness and distress

67. A 7-year old patient is diagnosed with acute glomerulonephritis. Which of the following should the nurse recommend in terms of diet?

A. regular diet, restricted sodium

B. low sodium, high protein diet

C. low sodium, low protein diet

D. low potassium, low protein diet

68. A patient was diagnosed with tuberculosis (TB) has been on isolation for 4 weeks. The isolation

precaution may be removed if this condition is met:

A. no adventitious breath sounds noted

B. absence of infiltrates in a repeat chest X-ray

C. negative sputum AFB after finishing the course of TB regimen

D. Anti-TB medication therapy including INH has been administered for the last 4 weeks

69. A patient is recently diagnosed with congestive heart failure. The nurse auscultates the lungs and notices crackling sounds on the bases of the lungs. The nurse should document this finding as:

A. Atelectasis

B. Rales

C. Rhonchi

D. Wheezing

70. The nurse coordinates with the dietitian regarding the diet requirement of a patient with renal failure. All of the following can be recommended, except:

A. potassium-rich foods

B. low sodium intake

C. carbohydrates-rich foods

D. a diet with eggs and dairy products

71. A newly diagnosed HIV-AIDS patient asks the nurse, "Can I infect other people with my sickness?" The nurse explains that HIV can be transferred in all of the following, except:

A. Touching or hugging

B. Saliva

C. Blood

D. Semen

72. A male stroke patient is newly diagnosed with depression due to current inability to perform activities of daily living on his own. What is the best way to initially communicate with the patient?

    A. Providing an information leaflet on depression

    B. Encouraging family to talk to the patient

    C. Using silence

    D. Using open-ended questions

73. A 93-year old patient is newly admitted due to pneumonia. To prevent disorientation of the patient, all of the following nursing interventions should be done except?

    A. Performing routine rounds

    B. Doing re-orientation with the patient every night

    C. Providing a night light

    D. Putting the bed rails up

74. Upon initial physical assessment, the patient says, "I find it difficult to distinguish scents when my eyes are closed." The nurse suspects that there might be a problem with which cranial nerve?

A. CN V

B. CN I

C. CN III

D. CN II

75. A 25-year old patient is admitted to the urgent care unit with asthma in exacerbation. Which of the following lung sounds should the nurse expect to hear upon auscultation?

A. Wheeze

B. Gurgle

C. Crackles

D. Pleural rub

76. A patient comes into the emergency unit with burns due to accidental electrocution. To determine the extent of the burn, the nurse examines the patient with which accurate assessment tools? Select two that apply.

A. Lund and Browder chart

B. Rule of Nines

C. Fitzpatrick's scale

D. GCS scale

77. A 45-year old patient is admitted with burn injuries extending to the muscles, bones, interstitial tissue, and some tendons. The health care provider classifies the burn injuries as:

  A. Subdermal burn
  B. Superficial burn
  C. Superficial partial thickness burn
  D. Full thickness burn

78. A tissue viability nurse conducts teaching on new staff on the risk factors of pressure sores. All of the following are risk factors associated with pressure injury, except?

  A. Advanced age
  B. Poor mobility
  C. Constipation
  D. Paralysis

79. Newborns exhibit several involuntary and unconscious responses known as reflexes. The physician documents,

"fencing reflex" on the newborn chart. This infant reflex is also known as:

A. Palmar reflex
B. Tonic neck reflex
C. Stepping reflex
D. Babinski reflex

80. A nurse manager wants to delegate some tasks to a staff nurse who has just graduated and requires mentoring for 2 months as per hospital protocol. Which of the following actions can be delegated to this member of the staff?

A. Suctioning of tracheostomy
B. Postmortem care
C. Taking vital signs
D. Evaluation of care plan

81. A post-vaginal surgery patient is transferred to the recovery room. In consideration of the patient's position during the surgery, the nurse should particularly assess for which of the following signs?

A. Arrhythmia

B. Biochemistry

C. Bowel sounds

D. Homan's sign

82. The nurse is doing her night rounds when she noticed that one of the patients admitted with pneumonia started to shiver. What is the first nursing intervention to be performed?

A. Inform the doctor that patient needs to be reviewed

B. Adjust the room temperature

C. Close the windows of the room

D. Apply warm blankets

83. A patient is moved to the recovery room following surgery. Which of the following assessment findings needs urgent nursing intervention?

A. temperature of 37.4 degrees Celsius

B. blood pressure of 120/70

C. pain score of 3 on a 10-point scale

D. urine output of 250 mL within the past 24 hours

84. The nurse enters the room of a post-surgery patient and found out that an internal organ is protruding 1.5 inches above the abdominal incision site. All the following nursing interventions are needed to be performed, except:

A. Perform observations and monitor for signs of shock

B. Place the patient in prone position to put pressure on the incision site

C. Inform the physician for an urgent review

D. Clean the site with normal saline and carefully place sterile dressing

85. A patient has not had any flatulence 48 hours after surgery. Upon auscultation, the nurse notices that there are no bowel sounds, and during inspection, the abdomen is distended. Which of the nursing interventions should the nurse do first?

A. Assist the patient to ambulate

B. Provide intravenous fluids

C. Administer enema

D. Encourage to drink at least 3000 liters of fluid per day

86. A post-operative patient is reviewed by the dietitian. The dietitian informs the nurse that the patient can now resume a solid, normal diet. Which of the following concerns should the nurse identify in relation to this change in diet?

A. Patient does not pass stool within 48 hours of resuming solid diet

B. Patient passes excessive flatulence

C. Patient does not pass stool within 12 hours of resuming solid diet

D. Patient refuses to eat solid food and wants a soup-based diet

87. An elderly female patient is diagnosed with a hip fracture following a fall in the bathroom. She rates her pain as 9 out of 10 and asks the nurse for pain relief. The pain can be described as:

A. Referred

B. Visceral

C. Phantom

D. Deep somatic

88. A nurse wants to delegate some tasks to a nursing assistive personnel. Which of the following can be delegated to this member of the staff?

A. Administering over-the-counter drugs for pain relief
B. Creating a care plan
C. Asking the patient to rate the level of pain on a 10-point scale basis
D. Asking the patient his/her medication history

89. A patient asks the nurse for acetaminophen (Tylenol) for pain relief. The nurse should question the order for acetaminophen if the patient has past medical history of:

A. Aspirin allergy
B. Gastric bleeding
C. Occasional alcohol drinking
D. Hepatitis B

90. A pancreatic cancer patient asks for pain relief due to severe abdominal pain, with a pain rating of 10 out 10. Before giving the prescribed Morphine IV to the patient, what should the nurse do first?

A. Monitor the heart rate
B. 6Check the respiratory status
C. Teach the patient deep breathing exercises
D. Query the order with the doctor who prescribed it

91. A patient is complaining of severe lower back pain. The nurse gives 60mg of codeine by mouth. The nurse should reassess the level of pain in:

A. 30 minutes
B. 10 minutes
C. 4 hours
D. 1 hour

92. A patient is admitted with a high risk for thrombophlebitis. Which of the following anti-

inflammatory drugs may be used to stop platelet aggregation in this patient?

A. Celecoxib

B. Aspirin

C. Indomethacin

D. Ibuprofen

93. The nurse assesses a newly admitted patient in the respiratory unit. Which of the following breath sounds of the patient should the nurse suspect as needing the most urgent medical intervention?

A. Wheezes

B. Stridor

C. Rhonchi

D. Crackles

94. A senior nurse is mentoring a nursing student on how to take vital signs properly. The nurse tells the student that an apical pulse needs to be observed on a patient who is:

A. Elderly with antidepressant medication

B. Infant with no history of congenital defect

C. Athlete with radial pulse of 60 bpm

D. Feverish with radial pulse of 90bpm

95. A nurse is attempting to accomplish a falls risk assessment on a newly admitted patient. All of the following can increase the risk for fall, except?

A. Skin biopsy

B. Use of walking prosthesis

C. History of dizziness

D. Orthostatic hypotension

96. The tissue viability nurse notices that a stroke patient has lost the uppermost layer of skin on one of the buttocks. The nurse should document this finding as:

A. Pressure ulcer

B. Excoriation

C. Abrasion

D. Maceration

97. In the history of nursing in the United States, the initial programs for nurse trainees were in conjunction with which kind of institution?

A. Religious orders
B. Civil service
C. Hospitals and town clinics
D. Military

98. Nursing is a discipline as well as a profession. Which of the following best supports this statement?

A. Having a scope of practice
B. Practice evidenced by scientific research
C. Creation of professional nursing boards and organizations
D. Establishment of nursing standards of care

99. An elderly patient appears pale and weak and has had 5 episodes of watery loose stools. The nurse recognizes that the patient is at risk of fluid volume deficit. All the following nursing interventions should be performed by the nurse, except:

A. Ask the doctor to prescribe intravenous fluids

B. Administer anti-diarrheal medication

C. Encourage the patient to increase oral fluid intake if not contraindicated

D. Re-position the patient to semi-Fowler's

100. A nurse administers the first dose of Co-amoxiclav 1.2 G intravenously to a patient with respiratory tract infection. After 10 minutes, the patient starts to develop hives. This reaction can be considered as:

A. Synergism

B. Allergy

C. Tolerance

D. Expected Reaction

101. Term to describe the reactivation and recurrence of pronounced symptoms of a disease:

A. Remission

B. Acute

C. Exacerbation

D. Urgent

102. A type of illness characterized by periods of remission and exacerbation:

    A. Emergent

    B. Acute

    C. Chronic

    D. Urgent

103. A person or animal, who is without signs of illness but harbors pathogen within their body and can be transferred to another:

    A. Carrier

    B. Fomite

    C. Agent

    D. None of the above

104. Removing pathogens but not their spores are an example of which process?

    A. Disinfection

    B. Sterilization

    C. Auto Claving

D. None of the above

105. Contact transmission of infectious organism in the hospital is usually cause by?

    A. Ventilation System

    B. Spread by cross contamination by hands of health care workers

    C. Using clean instruments not sterilized

    D. None of the above

106. Transmission occurs when an infected person sneezes, coughs or laugh that is usually projected at a distance of 3 feet:

    A. Fomite transmission

    B. Vector transmission

    C. Droplet transmission

    D. All of the above

107. The single most important procedure that prevents cross contamination and infection:

    A. Washing Hands

    B. Sterilizing

C. Cleaning with bleach

D. None of the above

108. A patient in the emergency room crashed on his scooter and sustained multiple lacerations. Tetanus toxoid Immunoglobulin was given as ordered by the provider. What immunity does tetanus toxoid Immunoglobulin give?

    A. Artificial passive immunity

    B. Artificial active immunity

    C. Natural passive immunity

    D. Natural active immunity

109. A client has been diagnosed with impetigo. What precaution is used for this patient?

    A. Airborne precautions

    B. Bloodborne precautions

    C. Droplet precautions

    D. Contact precautions

110. When applying sterile gloves, what should the nurse glove first?

A. Dominate hand

B. Non dominate hand

C. Either hand

D. All of the above

Fundamentals Review Questions with Answers and Rationales

NCLEX: Fundamentals of Nursing

1. An elderly patient is admitted under your care and exhibits an impaired gait. To reduce the risk of falls, to which member of the healthcare team should you refer this patient?

    E. Nurse practitioner

    F. Podiatrist

    G. Occupational therapist

    H. Physical therapist

Answer: D

Rationale: Physical therapists are licensed professionals that perform assessment, planning, implementation and evaluation of a patient's ability to function in terms of balance, mobility, gait, strength, range of motion, and coordination.

2. Your hospital uses the SBAR reporting system to relay information between the members of the healthcare team. Which of the following includes the correct elements of SBAR?

E. Signs and Symptoms, Basic patient information, Action, and Reaction

F. Situation, Background, Action, and Recommendation

G. Situation, Background, Assessment, and Recommendation

H. Signs and Symptoms, Background, Action, and Reaction

Answer: C

Rationale:

Situation includes the patient's diagnosis, current complaint, and care plan

Background includes the past medical history, DNR status, current medications, and diagnostic results

Assessment includes observations, signs and symptoms and mental status

Recommendation includes pending or proposed diagnostic tests and changes in care plan

3. A patient complains of having a burning sensation and pain on the peripheral cannula site. You observe that there

is warmth, redness, swelling and tenderness on the area. The patient is likely to be suffering from:

E. Phlebitis

F. Infiltration

G. Hematoma

H. Infection

Answer: A

Rationale: Phlebitis is evidenced by erythema (redness), swelling, tenderness and burning pain. Infiltration causes swelling but no erythema. Infection is unlikely as there is no pus or drainage. It is also rot hematoma as there is no localized bleeding.

4. A healthcare provider is about to render personal care to a 77-year old patient. It is important to use long and firm strokes and start from distal to proximal areas in order to:

E. Preserve the skin integrity

F. Reduce the risk of blood clot

G. Increase venous blood return

H. Promote vasoconstriction

Answer: C

Rationale: Long, firm strokes going from distal to proximal areas help improve circulation by increasing the venous blood return. The technique does not promote vasoconstriction, reduce the risk of blood clot or preserve the skin integrity.

5. A terminal patient under your care had peacefully died 10 minutes ago. While you prepare to inform the patient's family of the event, it is important to note which of the following five stages of death and dying according to Kubler-Ross?

    E. Bereavement, Crying, Depression, Regret, Denial

    F. Anger, Bargaining, Denial, Depression, Acceptance

    G. Bereavement, Anger, Denial, Depression, Acceptance

    H. Anger, Regret, Bereavement, Loneliness, Depression

Answer: B

Rationale: The five stages of death and dying according to Kubler-Ross include anger, bargaining, denial, depression, and acceptance. The patient and his/her significant others may go on different stages at different times.

6. A 65-year old patient is suspected to have hypoxia. Which of the following diagnostic tests should be done to verify this?

    E. Full blood count

    F. Biochemistry

    G. Arterial Blood Gas (ABG) Analysis

    H. Hemoglobin level

Answer: C

Rationale: ABG analysis is a test used to evaluate the exchange of blood gases in the lungs, thus providing an accurate information of the status of the patient's oxygenation.

7. A 35-year old patient is being monitored for adverse reactions to barbiturate therapy. One of these is considered as a major disadvantage of barbiturate therapy.

    E. Hepatotoxicity

    F. Drug dependence

    G. Reduced absorption

    H. Slow action

Answer: B

Rationale: With long-term use, barbiturates can cause a person to be dependent on them. A person with barbiturate dependence may experience withdrawal symptoms such as nausea, vomiting, and severe headache.

8. A 78 –year old female patient has severe difficulty of swallowing. The doctor and the dietitian agreed to prescribe enteral feeding for her. Which of the following nursing actions should be done when giving continuous enteral feeding?

    E. Warm the enteral feed formula using a microwave

    F. Elevate the head of the bed

    G. Ask the patient to lean on her left side

    H. Administer at a standard rate of 100 mL per hour

Answer: B

Rationale: Elevating the head of the bed minimizes the patient's risk of aspiration while on continuous feed. If there is a contraindication to elevate the head of the bed, position the patient to her right side. The formula feed should be at room temperature to avoid gastrointestinal upset. The rate of administration depends on the volume and duration as prescribed by the dietitian.

9. A post-mastectomy patient arrives in the surgical unit for continuity of care. After 4 hours, the nurse comes into the patient's room and suspects that she might be having shock as evidenced by:

E. Pale, dry, and warm skin

F. Urine output of 30 mL per hour

G. Respiratory rate of 17

H. Restlessness

Answer: D

Rationale: The earliest sign of shock is a change in mental status such as restlessness, irritability or anxiety due to the increase in the activity of the sympathetic nervous system that causes rapid secretion of epinephrine. Choices A, B, and C are all within normal range.

10. A nurse working in an outpatient unit witnesses a 65-year old male patient to faint and become unconscious. During rapid assessment, which pulse should the nurse palpate?

E. Femoral

F. Carotid

G. Radial

H. Brachial

Answer: B

Rationale: The carotid artery is the best one to palpate during a rapid assessment in order to assess the circulation of an unconscious adult patient. In infants, the brachial artery should be palpated. Other points of palpation may not be palpable in patients with circulatory problems.

11. A nurse is caring for a pregnant patient who is at a very high risk for a life-threatening situation while her baby is also at high risk for fetal death. Which of the following roles should the nurse prioritize?

E. Advocate

F. Coordinator of care

G. Case manager

H. Collaborator

Answer: A

Rationale: While all of these nursing roles are important for this patient, advocacy is the highest priority in this situation. The nurse should advocate for the wishes of the parents, as well as the wellbeing of the baby. It is important for the nurse to seek help from the hospital's ethics committee to resolve this ethical dilemma.

12. In the emergency room, a 44-year old male patient agrees to be admitted in the medical after the physician diagnosed him with lower respiratory tract infection. He sits on the wheelchair and the porter brings him to the ward. Which type of legal consent was exhibited?

    E. Explicit consent

    F. Opt-out consent

    G. Implicit consent

    H. Emergency consent

Answer: C

Rationale: When the patient agrees to be admitted, he gives the implicit consent of voluntary acute care hospitalization. Explicit consent usually happens when a patient signs a consent document, for instance, to undergo a surgical procedure.

13. A newly diagnosed Parkinson's patient suffers from hand tremors. She will need adaptive devices to help her cut food and eat her meals properly. The nurse can refer

this patient to which member of the multidisciplinary healthcare team?

  E. Physical therapist

  F. Occupational therapist

  G. Dietitian

  H. Nutritionist

Answer: B

Rationale: Occupational therapists are healthcare professionals that can assess, plan, implement, and evaluate a patient's functional ability to have the best possible independence level in terms of activities of daily living, such as eating, dressing, bathing, and grooming.

14. A 74-year old male patient with congestive heart failure was admitted in the Intensive Care Unit. After 10 days, his condition has stabilized and he is now to be transferred to the medical ward. Which of the following terms best describes this scenario?

  E. Critical pathway

  F. Continuity of Care

  G. Case Management

H. Cardiac protocol

Answer: B

Rationale: The scenario is an example of continuity of care, which involves a smooth, logical and timely transition to either a lower level or a higher level of care, depending of patient's changing needs.

15. A community health nurse is planning a presentation on the risk factors for cancer. Which of the following categories of risk factors is considered the most modifiable?

E. Lifestyle choices

F. External locus of control

G. Genetic predisposition

H. High risk behaviors

Answer: A

Rationale: Lifestyle choices are the most modifiable and correctable category of risk factors. These include smoking, excessive sun exposure, poor food choices, and alcohol abuse.

16. A nurse needs to relay important information to the patient's attending physician. Which of the following statements should be included in the "Assessment" part of SBAR?

E. The nurse tells the doctor that the patient's current diagnosis is ulcerative colitis.

F. The nurse informs the physician that the patient has 3 episodes of watery stools.

G. The nurse tells the doctor that the patient may benefit from additional IV fluids.

H. The nurse informs the physician that the stool culture is positive for C. difficile.

Answer B

Rationale: Using SBAR, the vital signs, symptoms, and patient's verbalizations are part of the "Assessment" of the nurse. Choice A can be included in "Situation", choice C is a "Recommendation", and Choice D is a "Background".

17. A post-surgical male patient is about to be discharged. The nurse shows the home medications that the patient needs to take and tells him the right doses and frequency for each drug. The nurse asks the patient to repeat the information back to her to assess his understanding. Which

of the following professional roles does the nurse perform in this scenario?

    E. Advocate

    F. Case manager

    G. Care giver

    H. Educator

Answer: D

Rationale: In this scenario, the nurse attempts to educate the patient about his home medications. The educator role of the nurse also involves the assessment of the patient's level of understanding before and after the teaching session.

18. A female patient is going to have a hysterectomy in the afternoon. She shows the early signs of heightened anxiety. Which of the following is the best response by the healthcare provider?

    E. "Here's a booklet on your procedure. Read it and let me know if you have any questions."

    F. "Would you like me to turn on the television to distract you while waiting for the surgery?"

    G. "What is bothering you regarding this surgery?

H. "Everything will be okay, so don't worry too much about it."

Answer: C

Rationale: Anxiety emerges when a person feels isolated, insecure, helpless, or hopeless. Encouraging the patient to talk about her worries and fears regarding the surgery will help reduce her level of anxiety. The nurse should exhibit a supportive role to help alleviate the anxiety.

19. A patient complains of abdominal pain. The nurse starts the assessment with which of the following examination techniques?

E. Percussion

F. Auscultation

G. Palpation

H. Inspection

Answer: D

Rationale: In performing a physical examination, inspection is the first step to perform. After inspection, auscultation needs to be done, as both palpation and percussion may influence the patient's bowel motility.

20. A patient starting on chemotherapy has recently had a central venous catheter inserted for optimal access. In checking the radiological report on the proper positioning of this catheter, the tip should be in the:

E. Subclavian vein

F. Superior vena cava

G. Basilica vein

H. Jugular vein

Answer: B

Rationale: The tip of the central venous catheter usually lies on either of the three sites: superior vena cava, right atrium, or inferior vena cava, as these three are involved in central venous circulation.

21. During the night shift, an 83-year old female patient complains of not being able to sleep. Which of the following nursing interventions should the nurse do first?

E. Assist the client with the use of sleep aids such as pillows, snacks, back rubs, and a change of room temperature as needed.

F. Ask the physician to prescribe a sleeping medication and administer it.

G. Educate the patient to perform deep breathing exercises, guided imagery, and relaxation techniques.

H. Assess the patient's sleeping patterns and record in her sleeping chart.

Answer: A

Rationale: Simple nursing interventions such as the provision of normal sleep aids should be performed first before administering any sleeping medication or doing more time-consuming or greater skills such as relaxation techniques. Assessment of the sleeping pattern is necessary but not urgently required in this situation.

22. A 45-year old male patient is rushed into the emergency room following a serious motor vehicle accident. Which of the following nursing actions should the nurse prioritize?

E. Administer pain relief

F. Use a pillow as a splint to the chest wall

G. Assess the patient's airway

H. Teach the patient to perform deep breathing exercises

Answer: C

Rationale: The first priority of the nurse is to assess the patency of the client's airway. The nurse should look for any obstruction, stridor, wheezing, or sternal retraction. The rest of the choices can be used by the nurse after performing an assessment.

23. A 66-year old female patient goes back to the surgical ward after having a tonsillectomy. After 2 hours, the patient exhibits signs of lethargy and sore throat. Which of the following positions should be encouraged?

    E. Side-lying

    F. High Fowler's

    G. Supine

    H. Semi Fowler's

Answer: A

Rationale: The side lying position is the best position to prevent the risk of blood aspiration from the surgical wound of a post-tonsillectomy patient. The other positions may increase the risk for aspirating blood and do not encourage enough oral drainage.

24. A nurse needs to conduct a client interview on the patient's past medical history and current medications. Which of the following is the most appropriate behavior during the interview?

E. Sit on the chair at the bedside of the client and use active listening

F. Ask the patient, "Why did you choose to be admitted this time?"

G. Use accurate medical terms when asking questions

H. Provide a medical interview form to the patient, and come back when he/she has already finished answering it

Answer: A

Rationale: It is important for the nurse to use active listening during a patient interview in order to record accurate information about the patient as well as assess any verbal and non-verbal cues that will help in the plan of care. The nurse should avoid using medical jargon as much as possible as the patient may not fully understand complex medical terms.

25. A 24-year old male patient is newly admitted in the medical ward and the nurse attempts to do an initial set of

vital signs for him. What is the best position of the patient for this assessment, considering that there are no contraindications?

E. Side-lying

F. Supine

G. Prone

H. Sitting upright

Answer: D

Rationale: If there are no contraindications, an upright sitting position is the best way to conduct an initial assessment. This position encourages full expansion of the lungs, as well as easier access to auscultate breath sounds. It also allows direct eye contact between the nurse and the patient to establish rapport.

26. The nurse is performing a physical assessment of a 44-year old colitis patient. Which of the following will the nurse auscultate for when using the diaphragm of the stethoscope?

E. Carotid bruits

F. Heart murmurs

G. Jugular venous hums

H. Bowel sounds

Answer: D

Rationale: The diaphragm of the stethoscope is used to auscultate high pitched sounds such as bowel sounds, as well as breath sounds. The bell, on the other hand, is used for low-pitched sounds, such as jugular venous hums, heart murmurs, and carotid bruits.

27. A 22-year old female patient's body mass index is calculated as 27. This BMI can be considered as:

E. Underweight

F. Overweight

G. Obese

H. Average

Answer: B

Rationale: In adults, the average BMI is between 20 and 25. A BMI if less than 20 means that the patient is underweight, while a BMI of 25 to 29.9 is considered overweight. Obese patients have a BMI of more than 30.

28. The nurse is identifying some possible nursing diagnoses for a 32-year old post mastectomy patient. Which of the following models can she use to perform this?

Select all that apply

E. Gordon's functional health patterns

F. Body systems model

G. Maslow's hierarchy of needs

H. Head-to-toe physical assessment form

Answer: A and C

Nursing diagnoses require holistic models to ensure that the patient is being examined as a whole, not in parts. Holistic models include Gordon's functional health patterns and Maslow's hierarchy of needs. Body systems models and Head-to-toe assessments focus on the identification of disease or physiological needs.

29. A patient who is morbidly obese will benefit from reducing the pressure from the skin folds using which of the following nursing interventions?

E. Applying barrier cream on the skin

F. Using a sheepskin mattress protector

G. Aiding the skin folds with towels

H. Keeping the linens wrinkle free

Answer: D

Rationale: Keeping the linens wrinkle free helps reduce the pressure that is created by the skin folds in a morbidly obese patient. Sheepskin mattress cover is not recommended. Using towels in between skin folds will relieve the pressure of rubbing. A barrier cream Is useful when there is incontinence.

30. A nurse is doing a physical assessment of an 82-year old female patient. The assessment revealed that she has all of the following secondary defenses against infection, except:

E. Swelling of lymph nodes

F. Intact skin

G. Pus on the infected wound

H. Fever

Answer: B

Rationale: The secondary defense mechanism of the body against an infection include the use of immune cells (as evidenced by pus on the wound), lymph nodes, and fever (to re-establish homeostasis). One of the primary defenses against infections is an intact skin.

31. A patient is recovering from a massive stroke and exhibits signs of difficulty of swallowing. The nurse needs to refer this patient to which member of the multidisciplinary healthcare team?

    E. Physical therapist

    F. Speech therapist

    G. Respiratory therapist

    H. Occupational therapist

Answer: B

Rationale: Speech and language therapists are professional healthcare workers who specialize in assisting the patient who have speech disturbances and difficulty of swallowing.

32. A 50-year old male patient has an established ascending colostomy. Before changing the colostomy bag, the nurse assesses the site and is likely to inform the physician about which of the following findings?

    E. The colostomy delivered liquid feces.

F. There is redness on the skin after immediately removing the appliance.

G. The stoma is raised to ½ inch above the abdomen.

H. The stoma has a purplish color.

Answer: D

Rationale: The normal color of an established stoma is dark pink to beefy red. It is normal for it to be slightly extending above the abdomen, as well as having redness on the skin after immediate removal of the colostomy appliance. Ascending colostomy with liquid stools is within normal range. Having a purplish stoma color requires immediate intervention of the physician as well as the stoma nurse.

33. A 49-year old female patient calls for a nurse in her room and complains of abdominal pain and is also worried about her stools. Upon assessment, the nurse will suspect of intestinal bleeding with which of the following stool characteristics?

E. Watery and greenish stools

F. Yellow blobs of stool floating in the toilet

G. Soft and black, tarry stools

H. Pencil shaped brown stools

Answer: C

Rationale: Blood in the gastrointestinal tract results to black and tarry stools. Yellow, fat-containing stools might indicate malabsorption. Watery stools might indicate C.difficile diarrhea, and pencil shaped stools might be a sign of rectal obstruction.

34. An elderly female patient had a hip surgery following a fall and now shows signs of fecal incontinence. The nurse can use which of the following nursing diagnoses? Select all that apply.

E. Disturbed Body Image

F. Risk for deficient fluid volume

G. Bowel incontinence

H. Risk for impaired skin integrity

Answer: A, C, and D

Rationale: The patient may not be at risk for deficient fluid volume if there are no signs of diarrhea associated with fecal incontinence. Bowel incontinence is the best nursing diagnosis for this patient. She might have a disturbed body image if she was previously well enough to control her fecal elimination. She is also at risk for impaired skin integrity due to increased skin moisture from fecal material post surgery.

35. A nurse manager shows a new male nurse around the unit and shows the different equipment used for personal care. She tells him that a fracture bedpan can be used for which kind of patient?

E. On bedrest

F. Dementia

G. Morbidly obese

H. Has a spinal cord injury

Answer: D

Rationale: A fracture bedpan is smaller than standard bedpans and has a low back or flat end that helps support a patient with spinal cord injury or hip fracture.

36. A female nurse is discussing effective ways to manage constipation with a 65-year old patient. She tells the patient to avoid excessive straining when trying to pass stools to prevent:

E. Fecal impaction

F. Dysrhythmia

G. Incontinence

H. Hemorrhoids

Answer: B

Rationale: Excessive straining when attempting to eliminate stools usually involves holding the breath while bearing down. This may increase both intracranial and intrathoracic pressures, and eventually cause respiratory difficulties and cardiac dysrhythmias. Hemorrhoids may also result from this maneuver, although these are not the primary rationale for avoiding it as they are not life-threatening.

37. The nurse instructs the patient on how to properly collect a stool sample for a stool culture test. Which of the following should be included in this teaching?

E. The stool specimen must not be mixed with any drop of urine.

F. The sample bottle must be filled to the top.

G. Eating a lot of meat prior to stool collection is optimal.

H. If the stool is red in color, it is unacceptable.

Answer: A

Rationale: It is ideal for the stool specimen not to be contaminated by urine to get the most accurate results. The sample does not necessarily need to fill the whole bottle. Eating a lot of protein such as poultry, red meat or fish prior to testing may alter the results. The color of the stool does not have to be brown. A red stool may indicate bleeding in the gastrointestinal tract.

38. A nurse notices that the patient with chronic obstructive pulmonary disease (COPD) has bluish discoloration of the lips. What the accurate term that she should use when documenting this finding?

E. Dyspnea

F. Cyanosis

G. Hypoxia

H. Hypoxemia

Answer: B

Rationale: Cyanosis is the bluish discoloration of the mucous membranes, including the lips. Dyspnea is a term used to describe difficulty of breathing, while hypoxia and hypoxemia require further data on the patient's oxygenation.

39. A patient with upper respiratory tract infection is unable to remove his phlegm on his own. The nurse uses a nasopharyngeal suction using which appropriate technique?

E. Hyper-oxygenate the patient with 100% oxygen for 30 minutes

F. Rotate the catheter while suctioning

G. Suction intermittently while inserting the catheter

H. Lubricate the catheter generously with petroleum jelly

Answer: B

The proper technique of applying nasopharyngeal suctioning is to rotate the catheter to prevent the pulling of tissue into the catheter tip's opening. It is important to use only water based lubricants. The suction should not be applied while inserting the catheter to avoid trauma. Hyper-oxygenation is usually recommended for intubated or tracheostomy patients and should only last for a few minutes prior to suctioning.

40. A patient who has chronic pulmonary disease needs teaching on how to use the incentive spirometer properly.

Which of the following statements indicate correct understanding of this procedure?

E. "I can use the device three times a day before and after meals. "

F. "I should breathe in fast and breathe out as fast and hard as I can."

G. "I must inhale in a slowly and steady manner in order to keep the balls up."

H. "I should use soapy water to clean the device every week."

Answer: C

The proper use of incentive spirometer includes using slow and steady inhalations, with 5 to 10 repetitions every 1 to 2 hours. It is important to clean only the mouthpiece and wipe clean every after use.

41. A nurse conducts health teaching on the patient who is post hip replacement surgery. She tells the patient that the best way to implement deep breathing exercises includes which of the following?

E. Use diaphragmatic breathing with pursed lips 5 to 10 times a day

F. Perform forceful coughing 3 to 5 times a day

G. Conduct deep breathing exercises 1 hour before
   and after meals

H. Use huff coughing every 2 hours or as the patient
   can tolerate

Answer: D

Rationale: Huff coughing facilitates mobilization of
secretions while keeping the airways open. Post-operative
patients may be unable to do normal and forceful
coughing. It is ideal to do huff coughing before and after
meals or as often as every 2 hours.

42. A 6-year old patient requires tracheostomy care. before
starting to perform the procedure the first thing that the
nurse should do includes:

E. Clean the incision site

F. Ask the patient to raise his right hand if he feels any
   pain or distress while doing the procedure

G. Change the twill tape that holds the tracheostomy
   in place

H. Check how tied the knot and ties are

Answer: B

Rationale: Before starting the tracheostomy care, the nurse and the patient should agree with a means of communication when there is any pain or distress during the procedure. The twill tape should be changed after performing the care of the tracheostomy.

43. The patient verbalizers, "I feel short of breath when I'm lying down, but I seem to feel better when I sit upright." The nurse recognizes that the patient is experiencing:

    E. Acapnea

    F. Orthopnea

    G. Hypernea

    H. Dyspnea

Answer: B

Rationale: The patient has difficulty of breathing that is noticeable when changing positions. The appropriate term for this respiratory problem is orthopnea.

44. A 44-year old patient is diagnosed with acute bronchitis. The physician ordered to start corticosteroid therapy. The nurse tells the patient that corticosteroids will help:

    E. Facilitate coughing

F. Achieve bronchodilaticn

G. Reduce the inflammation of the airways

H. Avoid contracting a respiratory infection

Answer: C

Rationale: Corticosteroid therapy is prescribed with the main aim of reducing the inflammation of the airways. The other choices are not achieved by using corticosteroids.

45. A male patient with chronic pulmonary disease is unable to expectorate phlegm on her own. The nurse plans to do postural drainage and percussion to help him. When is the best time for the nurse to do this procedure?

E. After breakfast so the patient has energy

F. Before lunch with an empty stomach

G. 30 minutes after hyper-oxygenating the patient

H. After dinner so the patient can sleep right after the procedure

Answer: B

Rationale: The optimal time for the nurse to perform postural drainage and percussion is before meal time to minimize the discomfort of the patient. The patient may ingest some of the secretions, which leave an unpleasant taste in the mouth and might cause nausea and vomiting.

46. A male elderly patient is prescribed with intravenous therapy and requires a new peripheral cannula to be inserted on his forearm. Because of a previous difficulty in cannulation, the nurse decides to apply a warm compress on the forearm prior to doing the procedure. The nurse explains to the patient that the heat:

    E. Alleviates the discomfort

    F. Minimizes the muscle spasms

    G. Increases circulation

    H. Prevents hemorrhage

Answer: C

Rationale: Applying warm compress transfers heat on the skin surface and this helps promote the dilation of the vein by increase the blood flow to the desired area of cannulation. On the other hand, cold compress facilitates vasoconstriction.

47. The doctor refers a newly admitted 85-year old female patient to chest physiotherapy service with the goal of

expectorating thick phlegm using vibration and percussion. With the correct knowledge of the patient's past medical history, the nurse needs to question this order if the patient has:

E. Cystic fibrosis

F. Osteoporosis

G. Emphysema

H. Bronchitis

Answer: B

Rationale: Osteoporosis is the abnormal loss of the mass and strength of bones, common in the elderly and female adults. A patient with osteoporcsis may suffer from fractures if vibration and percussion of the chest are performed. Therefore, the nurse should question the order to promote patient safety and discuss the concern with the doctor and the rest of the multidisciplinary team.

48. A male patient calls the nurse and complains of difficulty of breathing. He is already receiving oxygen via nasal cannula while lying in bed. What is the first nursing intervention that must be performed?

E. Notify the physician

F. Check for any secretions and suction as needed

G. Assist the patient to a Fowler's position

H. Assess the oxygen levels using a pulse oximeter

Answer: C

Rationale: The first priority of the nurse is to assist the patient to a Fowler's position in order to optimize the patient's breathing and allow for a better lung expansion. After positioning the patient, the nurse then assesses the patient's level of oxygenation, performs suctioning as needed, and notifies the physician to recommend an increase in oxygen therapy level if not contraindicated.

49. An 89-year old nursing home resident gets admitted to the medical unit after 4 days of refusing to eat or drink. Which of the following findings should the health care provider expect?

E. Swollen mucous membranes

F. Distention of the jugular veins

G. High blood pressure

H. Weak and rapid pulse

Answer: D

Rationale: A patient who has not eaten or drunk anything for a few days is likely suffering from fluid volume deficit, which is evidenced by a weak and rapid pulse. The other options are findings for a patient with fluid volume excess.

50. A 60-year old male patient comes into the emergency unit with nausea and dizziness, and has had 5 episodes of watery, loose stools. Upon assessment, the patient verbalizes, "I've been having leg cramps since last night and I feel so weak." Which nursing intervention must be done first?

    E. Administer an anti-emetic drug.

    F. Review the patient's serum electrolytes.

    G. Start an intravenous drip.

    H. Ask the doctor to prescribe pain medication for leg cramping.

Answer: B

Rationale: The nurse should check the results of the blood test of the patient, particularly the serum electrolytes, as leg cramping and lethargy are signs of low potassium levels. When a patient has diarrhea, electrolytes are eliminated with water from the body. After reviewing the electrolytes, the nurse can then perform the other options as above.

51. A nurse teaches the patient on proper breathing exercises. When teaching the patient about the purpose of pursed lip breathing, the nurse should inform the patient that it helps:

 E. Lower intrathoracic pressure

 F. Facilitate more effective coughing

 G. Help keep the airways open

 H. Allow the patient to expectorate phlegm

Answer: C

Rationale: Pursed lip breathing aims to maintain open airways by means of creating a resistance of air flow out of the lungs, thus prolonging exhalation. This breathing technique includes deep inhalations with slightly closed lips and long expirations.

52. A senior staff nurse teaches a student nurse on the principles of precautions in the medical unit. The nurse tells the student to use clean gloves in which of the following nursing interventions for a non-isolated patient?

E. Performing oral care

F. Doing a back rub

G. Assisting the client in feeding

H. Providing hair care

Answer: A

Rationale: A non-isolated patient means that it is safe for the healthcare provider to perform non-invasive procedures such as back rubs, massage, hair care, assistance in mobility, and feeding. However, oral care may put the nurse at risk as oral secretions are involved in this procedure, so there is a need for protection by using clean gloves.

53. A 75-year old male patient is admitted due to severe dehydration, diarrhea and vomiting. Which is the best method of assessing the patient's temperature?

E. Axillary

F. Oral

G. Radial

H. Tympanic

Answer D

Rationale: In assessing the temperature of this patient, the most accessible and less risky method for the nurse is to do the procedure through the ear, also known as tympanic temperature.

54. Upon doing baseline observations, the nurse records the respiratory rate of the patient as 25 respirations per minute in room air. Which of the following terms is appropriate in documenting this finding?

    E. Hyperpyrexia

    F. Tachypnea

    G. Tachycardia

    H. Arrhythmia

Answer: B

Rationale: Tachypnea means rapid respirations or higher than normal respiratory rate. Tachycardia means rapid heart rate. Hyperpyrexia means an increased level of temperature, and arrythmia means irregularity in heart rate.

55. A nurse is doing a neurological examination on a newly admitted patient. Using the Glasgow Coma Scale, the patient scores 15 out of 15. This means that the patient is:

E. Unconscious

F. Semi-conscious

G. Fully alert

H. Has a minor brain injury

Answer: C

Rationale: The Glasgow Coma Scale is a 15-point neurological assessment tool. A score of 15 out of 15 means that the patient has no brain injury or damage and is fully alert.

56. A patient with a Glasgow Coma Scale (GCS) score of 5 requires frequent mouth care. Before starting the procedure, the nurse should position the patient:

E. Trendelenburg

F. Lithotomy

G. Fowler's

H. Side lying

Answer: D

Rationale: A GCS score of 5 out 15 indicates that the patient is likely unconscious. To reduce the risk of aspiration while performing mouth care, the patient is best positioned on his side.

57. A 92-year old patient is newly admitted to the medical-surgical unit. Upon assessment, the nurse indicates that the patient is at high risk for falls because of all of the following factors except:

E. History of allergic rhinitis

F. Advanced age

G. Recent hip fracture

H. Use of a cane

Answer: A

Rationale: Falls risk assessment involves considering different factors such as age, recent injury, trauma, or surgery, related past medical history, and the use of mobility devices. Having a history of allergic rhinitis does not increase this patient's falls risk.

58. A 36-year old female patient comes into the emergency unit with complaints of nausea, vomiting, abdominal cramping, and watery stools. The nurse asks the patient some questions regarding any recent food intake. Which of

the following phases of nursing process does this scenario show?

E. Assessment

F. Diagnosis

G. Planning

H. Implementation

Answer A

Rationale: The nurse is attempting to gain information about the patient's food intake, which might be the cause of the signs and symptoms of the patient. This data collection is part of the assessment phase of the nursing process.

59. A medical-surgical nurse wants to apply Orem's theory in the nursing plan of care for a female patient with severe pulmonary disease. Which of the following can the nurse include in the care plan?

E. Love and belongingness

F. Physiological needs

G. Maintenance of sufficient intake of air

H. Self-perception

Answer: C

Rationale: The Self-care Theory of Dorothea Orem involves providing nursing care to achieve an optimal level of self-care in order for the patient to effectively function at home. This includes ways on how this pulmonary patient can maintain sufficient intake of air. The other choices are included in the Hierarchy of Needs by Abraham Maslow.

60. An elderly patient with full mental capacity refuses an injection, but the nurse administers the injection anyway as he/she thinks the patient needs it urgently. The nurse has committed:

    E. Malpractice

    F. Negligence

    G. Assault and battery

    H. None of the above

Answer: C

Rationale: The patient is of advanced age but with full mental capacity, which means he/she is capable of making healthcare decisions on his/her own. On the other hand, the nurse forces to administer the injection without the consent of the patient. This can be considered as assault, which is the threat or attempt to touch or injure another person. The situation is also an example of battery, which means the touching of another person against the law (that is, without consent).

61. A 25-month old pediatric patient comes into the emergency unit with fever, irritability, dry lips,

and watery loose stools. The mother said that the child has had 3 episodes of water loose stools

since the previous night. After assessing the patient, the nurse should prioritize which of the

following interventions?

A. Check the skin turgor

B. Obtain venous access

C. Weight the patient

D. Administer anti-diarrhea medication

Answer: B

Rationale: The pediatric patient is showing signs of dehydration. The nurse should prioritize

obtaining venous access and administering intravenous fluids as prescribed by the physician. Options

A and C are part of the assessment. Option D is a recommended intervention, but not the highest priority.

62. Upon performing a physical assessment of a newly admitted female patient, the patient shows a positive Homan's sign. Which of the following nursing interventions is the highest priority of the nurse?

A. Promote patient's skin integrity

B. Promote venous circulation

C. Maintain patency of the airways

D. Improve the balance of fluids and electrolytes

Answer: B

Rationale: Homan's sign is a characteristic sign of patients suffering from deep vein thrombosis (DVT). It is elicited by means of dorsiflexion of the ankle, resulting to calf pain. In this case, the nurse should promote good venous circulation of the patient.

63. A terminally ill cancer patient tells the nurse, "I am so afraid. Everyday my life seems to go downhill" The nurse

responds, "Tell me more about how you're feeling." What kind of therapeutic technique is being used?

A. Sympathy

B. Exploring

C. Focusing

D. Acknowledgement

Answer: B

Rationale: One of the most effective therapeutic techniques for communication is exploring, which gives the patient more time to express her thoughts, feelings, and fears, while the nurse is able to gain more information in order to create a better plan of care for the patient, as in this scenario.

64. An 89-yearold male patient with stage IV lung cancer is about to start on chemotherapy. He tells the nurse, "I don't actually want to have chemotherapy, but my children really want me to get this treatment." The nurse should assume which of the following professional roles to protect this patient?

A. Client advocate

B. Care provider

C. Educator

D. Counselor

Answer: A

Rationale: The nurse needs to assume the professional role of a client advocate to protect the

patient's wish of not starting treatment by means of further exploring the issues with the patient,

physician, and other important members of his healthcare team.

65. A burn patient comes into the medical unit and shows signs of dehydration and blood loss. To encourage hydration, which of the following intravenous fluids should the nurse recommend to the physician?

A. Lactated Ringer's solution

B. 0.9% Sodium Chloride

C. Dextrose 5% in Normal Saline

D. Dextrose 5% in Water

Answer: A

Rationale: Lactated Ringer's solution is the most appropriate type of intravenous fluid following a burn injury, surgery, or trauma that caused blood loss and dehydration.

66. An occupational health nurse is planning a short seminar on stress and its effect to employees. The nurse recognizes that stress can be described as all of the following except:

A. Stress may be physical, emotional, and/or spiritual.

B. Stress is a natural response and can be both adaptive and productive

C. Stress does not always lead to bodily damage

D. Stress always leads to feeling of hopelessness and distress

Answer: D

Answer: Stress does not always result to feeling of distress or hopelessness. Positive stress such as an upcoming wedding or having a new child may cause a person to develop feeling of joy and hope yet mixed with anxiety.

67. A 7-year old patient is diagnosed with acute glomerulonephritis. Which of the following should the nurse recommend in terms of diet?

A. regular diet, restricted sodium

B. low sodium, high protein diet

C. low sodium, low protein diet

D. low potassium, low protein diet

Answer: A

Rationale: Children with acute glomerulonephritis will benefit from low e or restricted sodium intake with regular diet to keep him/her nourished. Any progression to renal failure may result to the restriction of protein, potassium, and sodium.

68. A patient was diagnosed with tuberculosis (TB) has been on isolation for 4 weeks. The isolation precaution may be removed if this condition is met:

A. no adventitious breath sounds noted

B. absence of infiltrates in a repeat chest X-ray

C. negative sputum AFB after finishing the course of TB regimen

D. Anti-TB medication therapy including INH has been administered for the last 4 weeks

Answer: C

Rationale: The standard for removing respiratory precautions for a tuberculosis patient is when there are two negative sputum cultures for AFB, following the course of anti-tuberculosis regimen.

69. A patient is recently diagnosed with congestive heart failure. The nurse auscultates the lungs and notices crackling sounds on the bases of the lungs. The nurse should document this finding as:

A. Atelectasis

B. Rales

C. Rhonchi

D. Wheezing

Answer: B

Rationale: Rales are characterized by cracking sounds at the base of the lungs. Rhonchi are usually heard when the patient coughs and described as dry coarse sounds. Atelectasis is the term used for closure or collapse of the lungs. Wheezing is the sound heard when there is narrowing of air passages.

70. The nurse coordinates with the dietitian regarding the diet requirement of a patient with renal failure. All of the following can be recommended, except:

A. potassium-rich foods

B. low sodium intake

C. carbohydrates-rich foods

D. a diet with eggs and dairy products

Answer: A

Rationale: Patients diagnosed with renal failure need to have a positive nitrogen balance, so protein rich food such as eggs and dairy products are recommended. They also need energy, so a reasonably high caloric intake is necessary. The kidney damage requires the patient to have very low or restricted sodium intake. The patient should avoid potassium rich foods due to the reduced capacity of the kidneys in terms of the filtering and excretion of potassium.

71. A newly diagnosed HIV-AIDS patient asks the nurse, "Can I infect other people with my sickness?" The nurse explains that HIV can be transferred in all of the following, except:

    E. Touching or hugging

    F. Saliva

    G. Blood

H. Semen

Answer: A

Rationale: HIV can be transmitted through saliva, blood, semen, cerebrospinal fluid and other bodily fluids. Simple body contact such as hugging and touching does not transmit the virus.

72. A male stroke patient is newly diagnosed with depression due to current inability to perform activities of daily living on his own. What is the best way to initially communicate with the patient?

    E. Providing an information leaflet on depression

    F. Encouraging family to talk to the patient

    G. Using silence

    H. Using open-ended questions

Answer: D

Rationale: A person with depression may benefit from voicing out his fears, worries and anxieties. Although the other options can be applied to his plan of care, the initial way to communicate with the patient is to use open-ended questions to allow him to express his feelings.

73. A 93-year old patient is newly admitted due to pneumonia. To prevent disorientation of the patient, all of the following nursing interventions should be done except?

    E. Performing routine rounds

    F. Doing re-orientation with the patient every night

    G. Providing a night light

    H. Putting the bed rails up

Answer: D

Rationale: Elderly patients are at risk of disorientation, and would benefit with all of these nursing interventions, however, putting the bed rails up is least likely to contribute to this nursing goal as its main purpose is to prevent falls. The nurse needs to perform a bed rails assessment to check if the patient requires the bed rails to be up.

74. Upon initial physical assessment, the patient says, "I find it difficult to distinguish scents when my eyes are closed." The nurse suspects that there might be a problem with which cranial nerve?

    E. CN V

    F. CN I

    G. CN III

H. CN II

Answer: B

Rationale: The cranial nerve I is the olfactory nerve, which is responsible with the sense of smell, and sends signals to the brain, where the information about the scent is processed.

75. A 25-year old patient is admitted to the urgent care unit with asthma in exacerbation. Which of the following lung sounds should the nurse expect to hear upon auscultation?

E. Wheeze

F. Gurgle

G. Crackles

H. Pleural rub

Answer: A

Rationale: In patients with asthma in exacerbation, the airways become narrower. Wheezing sounds can be heard as air tries to pass through the constricted airways.

76. A patient comes into the emergency unit with burns due to accidental electrocution. To determine the extent of the burn, the nurse examines the patient with which accurate assessment tools? Select two that apply.

E. Lund and Browder chart

F. Rule of Nines

G. Fitzpatrick's scale

H. GCS scale

Answer: A and B

Rationale: Lund and Browder chart and Wallace's Rule of Nines tool are two assessment tools to determine the extent of burns, Lund and Browder chart is specifically the most accurate because it utilizes graphs that are age-dependent, therefore it can be also use for neonates and children,

77. A 45-year old patient is admitted with burn injuries extending to the muscles, bones, interstitial tissue, and some tendons. The health care provider classifies the burn injuries as:

E. Subdermal burn

F. Superficial burn

G. Superficial partial thickness burn

H. Full thickness burn

Answer: A

Rationale: Subdermal burn involves deep damage to the muscles, bones, interstitial tissue, and tendons. It is recommended to perform grafting, and the patient should be informed that scarring is to be expected.

78. A tissue viability nurse conducts teaching on new staff on the risk factors of pressure sores. All of the following are risk factors associated with pressure injury, except?

E. Advanced age

F. Poor mobility

G. Constipation

H. Paralysis

Answer: C

Rationale: All of the options are major risk factors for pressure ulcers, except for constipation, as it is likely to cause any pressure injury. On the other hand, diarrhea and incontinence may cause increase exposure to moisture and may contribute to the development of pressure sores.

79. Newborns exhibit several involuntary and unconscious responses known as reflexes. The physician documents, "fencing reflex" on the newborn chart. This infant reflex is also known as:

E. Palmar reflex

F. Tonic neck reflex

G. Stepping reflex

H. Babinski reflex

Answer: B

Rationale: Tonic neck reflex is another term for fencing reflex. This reflex is characterized as a postural reflex that usually disappears after 4 to 6 months of life.

80. A nurse manager wants to delegate some tasks to a staff nurse who has just graduated and requires mentoring for 2 months as per hospital protocol. Which of the following actions can be delegated to this member of the staff?

E. Suctioning of tracheostomy

F. Postmortem care

G. Taking vital signs

H. Evaluation of care plan

Answer: C

Rationale: A nurse who has just graduated can help the most with taking vital signs, as this is the most basic nursing action among all the options. The other options can be delegated to the nurse as he/ she gains mentoring and obtains more experience and training in the unit within the given timeframe.

81. A post-vaginal surgery patient is transferred to the recovery room. In consideration of the patient's position during the surgery, the nurse should particularly assess for which of the following signs?

A. Arrhythmia

B. Biochemistry

C. Bowel sounds

D. Homan's sign

Answer: D

Rationale: Vaginal surgeries require patients to assume the lithotomy position, making them at high risk for deep vein thrombosis (DVT). Homan's sign is the classical sign for DVT.

82. The nurse is doing her night rounds when she noticed that one of the patients admitted with

pneumonia started to shiver. What is the first nursing intervention to be performed?

A. Inform the doctor that patient needs to be reviewed

B. Adjust the room temperature

C. Close the windows of the room

D. Apply warm blankets

Answer: D

Rationale: Shivering is one of the earliest signs of hypothermia. The first nursing intervention for this is to apply warm blankets to control the temperature and shivering. The nurse can then perform temperature assessment the other options as necessary.

83. A patient is moved to the recovery room following surgery. Which of the following assessment findings needs urgent nursing intervention?

A. temperature of 37.4 degrees Celsius

B. blood pressure of 120/70

C. pain score of 3 on a 10-point scale

D. urine output of 250 mL within the past 24 hours

Answer: D

Rationale: Post-surgical patients require strict monitoring of input and output. The normal urinary output is at least 30 mL per hour, but the patient is only urinating about 10.5 mL per hour. The nurse should inform the physician urgently regarding this finding. The next nursing intervention is to offer pain relief to the patient. Options A and B are within normal range.

84. The nurse enters the room of a post-surgery patient and found out that an internal organ is protruding 1.5 inches above the abdominal incision site. All of the following nursing interventions are needed to be performed, except:

A. Perform observations and monitor for signs of shock

B. Place the patient in prone position to put pressure on the incision site

C. Inform the physician for an urgent review

D. Clean the site with normal saline and carefully place sterile dressing

Answer: B

Rationale: The patient is having wound evisceration, which is characterized by protrusion of organs. The patient should never be re-positioned to prone as it will worsen the situation. Instead, the nurse should encourage low Fowler's position with the knees bent. This will avoid tension in the abdomen. Then, the physician should examine the patient urgently.

85. A patient has not had any flatulence 48 hours after surgery. Upon auscultation, the nurse notices that there are no bowel sounds, and during inspection, the abdomen is distended. Which of the nursing interventions should the nurse do first?

A. Assist the patient to ambulate

B. Provide intravenous fluids

C. Administer enema

D. Encourage to drink at least 3000 liters of fluid per day

Answer: A

Rationale: Paralytic ileus is one of the complications of surgery. One of the signs of paralytic ileus is the failure to move bowels. The nurse should therefore prioritize ambulation of the patient while monitoring intake and output and maintaining NPO status.

86. A post-operative patient is reviewed by the dietitian. The dietitian informs the nurse that the patient can now resume a solid, normal diet. Which of the following concerns should the nurse identify in relation to this change in diet?

A. Patient does not pass stool within 48 hours of resuming solid diet

B. Patient passes excessive fatulence

C. Patient does not pass stool within 12 hours of resuming solid diet

D. Patient refuses to eat solid food and wants a soup-based diet

Answer: A

Rationale: The patient should pass stool within 48 hours following a resumption of solid normal diet. If the patient has not passed stool, he/ she might be experiencing constipation and must therefore need a doctor's review, dietary changes and/or medical intervention.

87. An elderly female patient is diagnosed with a hip fracture following a fall in the bathroom. She rates her pain as 9 out of 10 and asks the nurse for pain relief. The pain can be described as:

    E. Referred

    F. Visceral

    G. Phantom

    H. Deep somatic

Answer: C

Rationale: Pain that starts from bones, blood vessels, nerves, tendons, or ligaments can be identified as deep somatic pain. Hip fracture involves deep somatic pain originating from the bones.

88. A nurse wants to delegate some tasks to a nursing assistive personnel. Which of the following can be delegated to this member of the staff?

    E. Administering over-the-counter drugs for pain relief

F. Creating a care plan

G. Asking the patient to rate the level of pain on a 10-point scale basis

H. Asking the patient his/her medication history

Answer: C

Rationale: All of the options are tasks that should be done by a registered nurse and must not be delegated to a nursing assistive personnel, except for assessing the patient's pain based on a pain rating scale of 0 to 10. The finding should be relayed immediately to the nurse in charge of the patient. Assessment of drug history, care planning, and administering medications even if they are over-the-counter must be performed by the registered nurse.

89. A patient asks the nurse for acetaminophen (Tylenol) for pain relief. The nurse should question the order for acetaminophen if the patient has past medical history of:

E. Aspirin allergy

F. Gastric bleeding

G. Occasional alcohol drinking

H. Hepatitis B

Answer: D

Rationale: Acetaminophen, even in recommended doses, may cause severe liver damage in patients with hepatic disease, which includes Hepatitis B. Occasional alcohol drinking may not cause hepatotoxicity, but acetaminophen should be cautiously used in patients with regular alcohol intake.

90. A pancreatic cancer patient asks for pain relief due to severe abdominal pain, with a pain rating of 10 out 10. Before giving the prescribed Morphine IV to the patient, what should the nurse do first?

E. Monitor the heart rate

F. 6Check the respiratory status

G. Teach the patient deep breathing exercises

H. Query the order with the doctor who prescribed it

Answer: B

Rationale: Morphine belongs to a class of analgesics called opioids. These analgesics may cause respiratory depression, so it is important for the nurse to assess the respiratory status of the patient before and after administering morphine.

91. A patient is complaining of severe lower back pain. The nurse gives 60mg of codeine by mouth. The nurse should reassess the level of pain in:

E. 30 minutes

F. 10 minutes

G. 4 hours

H. 1 hour

Answer: D

Rationale: The peak concentration of oral codeine is 1 hour after administration. Therefore, the nurse should perform the evaluation of the effectiveness of the pain medication after an hour. The effectiveness of Intramuscular or intravenous codeine should be reassess after 10 minutes.

92. A patient is admitted with a high risk for thrombophlebitis. Which of the following anti-inflammatory drugs may be used to stop platelet aggregation in this patient?

E. Celecoxib

F. Aspirin

G. Indomethacin

H. Ibuprofen

Answer: B

Rationale: Aspirin is a nonsteroidal anti-inflammatory drug that can cause inhibition of platelet aggregation. It is common for doctors to prescribe a low dose aspirin for long term therapy to combat the risk of thrombophlebitis.

93. The nurse assesses a newly admitted patient in the respiratory unit. Which of the following breath sounds of the patient should the nurse suspect as needing the most urgent medical intervention?

E. Wheezes

F. Stridor

G. Rhonchi

H. Crackles

Answer: B

Rationale: If a patient has stridor, the nurse should suspect respiratory distress with a high possibility of obstructed airways. Wheezes are breath sounds that arise when air moves in narrowed airway. Rhonchi and crackles might indicate the presence of fluid in the lung.

94. A senior nurse is mentoring a nursing student on how to take vital signs properly. The nurse tells the student that an apical pulse needs to be observed on a patient who is:

E. Elderly with antidepressant medication

F. Infant with no history of congenital defect

G. Athlete with radial pulse of 60 bpm

H. Feverish with radial pulse of 90bpm

Answer: B

Rationale: Peripheral pulses might not be detected accurately in very young children (until 3 years of age) and infants, so apical pulse is the most accurate way to observe the patient's pulse rate. In addition to this, apical pulse rate needs to be taken on patients with irregular or weak pulses or on cardiac medication.

95. A nurse is attempting to accomplish a falls risk assessment on a newly-admitted patient. All of the following can increase the risk for fall, except?

E. Skin biopsy

F. Use of walking prosthesis

G. History of dizziness

H. Orthostatic hypotension

Answer: A

Rationale: Orthostatic hypotension, history of dizziness, recent fall, or fainting, use of walking prosthesis, advanced age, and use of cognition-altering medications can increase the risk for fall of a patient. Having a history of skin biopsy or most other minor surgical procedures will not contribute to the falls risk of the patient.

96. The tissue viability nurse notices that a stroke patient has lost the uppermost layer of skin on one of the buttocks. The nurse should document this finding as:

E. Pressure ulcer

F. Excoriation

G. Abrasion

H. Maceration

Answer: B

Rationale: Excoriation happens when the superficial layer of the skin is lost. This is usually due to the damage caused by digestive enzymes that are present in feces. It is not a pressure ulcer since there is no evidence of insufficient perfusion as well as tissue compression. Abrasion is caused by friction between the linen or clothing and the skin. Maceration is caused by long exposure to moisture and is described as softening of the skin.

97. In the history of nursing in the United States, the initial programs for nurse trainees were in conjunction with which kind of institution?

    E. Religious orders

    F. Civil service

    G. Hospitals and town clinics

    H. Military

Answer: A

Rationale: The American nurse trainees before and during the Civil War were already trained in religious orders prior to their nursing training, which was mainly conducted by the military.

98. Nursing is a discipline as well as a profession. Which of the following best supports this statement?

    E. Having a scope of practice

F. Practice evidenced by scientific research

G. Creation of professional nursing boards and organizations

H. Establishment of nursing standards of care

Answer: B

Rationale: Evidenced-based nursing grounded in scientific research is the defining characteristic of nursing as both a discipline and a profession. Standards of care, scope of practice, and professional nursing organizations are formulated and governed by scientific and technical knowledge based on sound research.

99. An elderly patient appears pale and weak and has had 5 episodes of watery loose stools. The nurse recognizes that the patient is at risk of fluid volume deficit. All of the following nursing interventions should be performed by the nurse, except:

E. Ask the doctor to prescribe intravenous fluids

F. Administer anti-diarrheal medication

G. Encourage the patient to increase oral fluid intake if not contraindicated

H. Re-position the patient to semi-Fowler's

Answer: D

Rationale: The patient is likely to be suffering from fluid volume deficit secondary to dehydration. All of the options are recommended nursing interventions for this client problem, except for re-positioning the patient as this does not contribute to the plan of care in this particular nursing diagnosis.

100. A nurse administers the first dose of Co-amoxiclav 1.2 G intravenously to a patient with respiratory tract infection. After 10 minutes, the patient starts to develop hives. This reaction can be considered as:

    E. Synergism

    F. Allergy

    G. Tolerance

    H. Expected Reaction

Answer: B

Rationale: The patient has developed an immunologic response to the first dose of the antibiotic. This can be described as a drug allergy, and is usually manifested by hives, rash or other skin changes, difficulty of breathing, or edema of one or more parts of the body. This is an adverse reaction that needs to urgent medical attention.

101. Term to describe the reactivation and recurrence of pronounced symptoms of a disease:

        E. Remission

        F. Acute

        G. Exacerbation

        H. Urgent

Answer: C

Rationale: Reactivation of symptoms of a disease is exacerbation

102. A type of illness characterized by periods of remission and exacerbation:

        E. Emergent

        F. Acute

        G. Chronic

        H. Urgent

Answer: C

Rationale: Illnesses with that have periods of remissions and exacerbations are termed chronic.

103. A person or animal, who is without signs of illness but harbors pathogen within their body and can be transferred to another:

      E. Carrier

      F. Fomite

      G. Agent

      H. None of the above

Answer: A

Rationale: Carrier is a person or animal who can harbor a pathogen without signs or symptoms.

104. Removing pathogens but not their spores are an example of which process?

      E. Disinfection

      F. Sterilization

      G. Auto Claving

      H. None of the above

Answer: A

Rationale: Disinfection will remove pathogens but not spores.

105. Contact transmission of infectious organism in the hospital is usually cause by?

  E. Ventilation System

  F. Spread by cross contamination by hands of health care workers

  G. Using clean instruments not sterilized

  H. None of the above

Answer: B

Rationale: Majority of contact transmission in the healthcare settings are by hands of the healthcare workers.

106. Transmission occurs when an infected person sneezes, coughs or laugh that is usually projected at a distance of 3 feet:

  E. Fomite transmission

  F. Vector transmission

  G. Droplet transmission

H. All of the above

Answer: C

Rationale: Droplet transmission occurs when bacteria or viruses travel on relatively large respiratory droplets that people sneeze, cough, drip, or exhale. Traveling only short distances before settling, usually less than 3 feet. The droplets are loaded with infectious particles. They can be spread directly if people are close enough to each other.

107. The single most important procedure that prevents cross contamination and infection:

        E. Washing Hands

        F. Sterilizing

        G. Cleaning with bleach

        H. None of the above

Answer: A

Rationale: Handwashing is most important procedure to prevent infection and cross contamination.

108. A patient in the emergency room crashed on his scooter and sustained multiple lacerations. Tetanus toxoid

Immunoglobulin was given as ordered by the provider. What immunity does tetanus toxoid Immunoglobulin give?

E. Artificial passive immunity

F. Artificial active immunity

G. Natural passive immunity

H. Natural active immunity

Answer: A

Rationale: Tetanus immune globulin creates an artificial passive immunity to the toxin of C. tetani

109. A client has been diagnosed with impetigo. What precaution is used for this patient?

E. Airborne precautions

F. Bloodborne precautions

G. Droplet precautions

H. Contact precautions

Answer: D

Rationale: Impetigo is typically spread from person to person through direct skin-to-skin contact. It is important to wash your hands after contact with patient with impetigo.

110. When applying sterile gloves, what should the nurse glove first?

      E. Dominate hand

      F. Non dominate hand

      G. Either hand

      H. All of the above

Answer: B

Rationale: Generally, applying sterile gloves to the non-dominate hand first is the standard procedure.